S I M P L Y

PILATES

S I M P L Y
PILATES

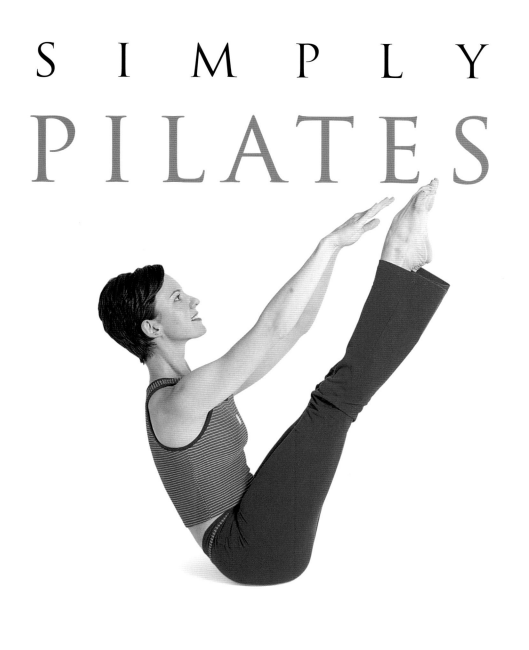

HINKLER
BOOKS

Editors: Bridget Blair & Robyn Sheahan-Bright
Creative Director: Sam Grimmer
Photography: Peter Wakeman
Design: Sam Grimmer

Published in 2002, Reprinted 2003 (twice),
Reprinted 2004 (four times), 2005
by Hinkler Books Pty Ltd
17-23 Redwood Drive
Dingley, VIC 3172, Australia
www.hinklerbooks.com

Printed and bound in China

ISBN 1 8651 5927 1

CONTENTS

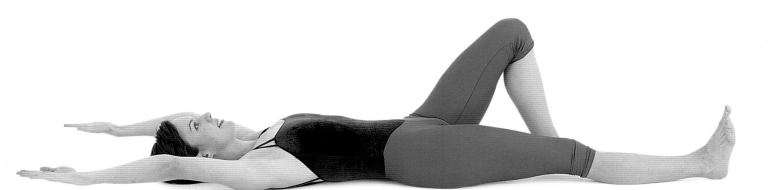

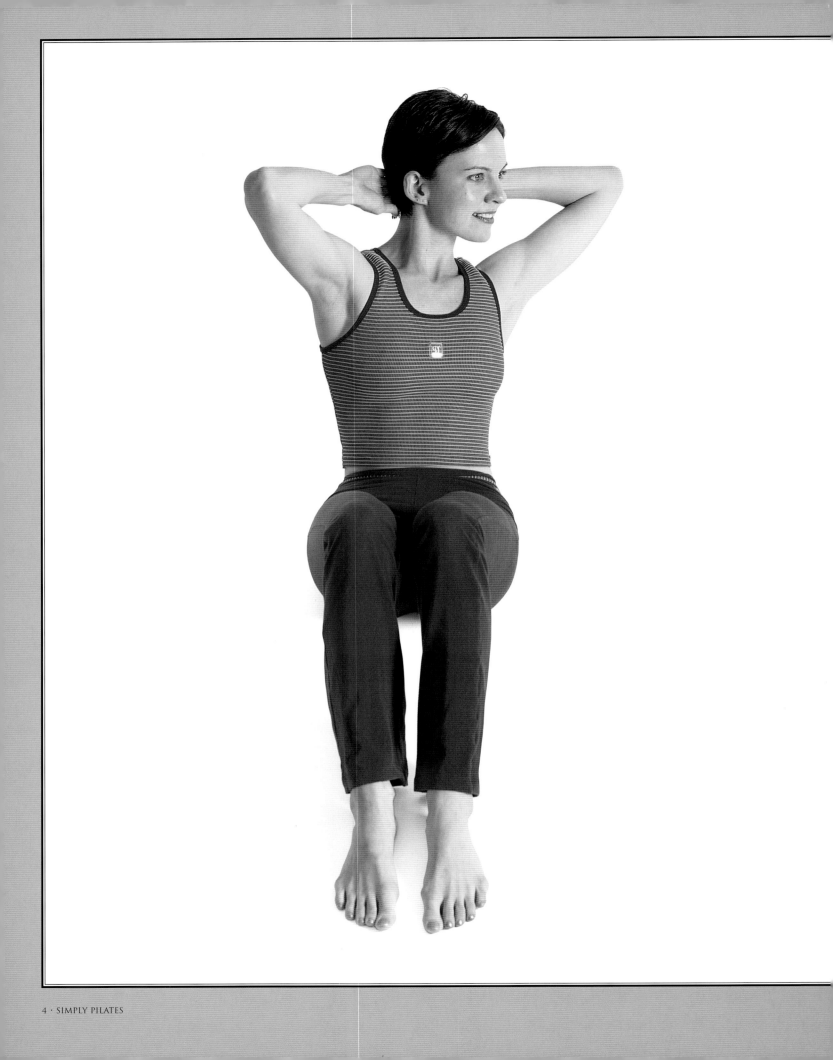

INTRODUCTION

The Pilates Method of exercising has become one of the most sought-after ways of maintaining one's fitness. Unique in its approach to working the body 'smart', not 'hard', it is renowned for achieving long-term physical benefits. It is endorsed by medical and fitness professionals in many countries for its ability to re-educate the body to move efficiently, improving the quality of an individual's daily activities.

Originally developed by German-born Joseph Pilates in the early 1900s, the technique has evolved, taking on various forms. During World War I, Pilates used his knowledge of strengthening the body to rehabilitate injured soldiers. He later operated his own exercise studio in New York, where many dancers, athletes and actresses were attracted to his training methods as a way to maintain a strong, supple and streamlined physique. Pilates called his method 'The Art of Contrology', though over the years it has taken on his own name of 'Pilates'. Its essential concept is to stretch and strengthen the body with heed to symmetry and alignment.

His movement system was designed to deliver the ultimate full-body workout in a gentle and effective manner, borrowing principles from various Eastern and Western exercise philosophies. He believed, foremost, that the mind controls the muscles and that endless repetitions of meaningless exercises do more harm than good. When exercising using Pilates' principles, the outcome is better posture, stronger and more flexible muscles, greater energy and an increased ability to cope with day-to-day stresses.

Pilates has become very popular with people in high-profile professions, such as dancers and actors, and has therefore become extremely 'trendy'. However, it is not, like some other exercise regimes, destined to become a transitory fad, since it is a highly disciplined form of exercise with a record of proven results.

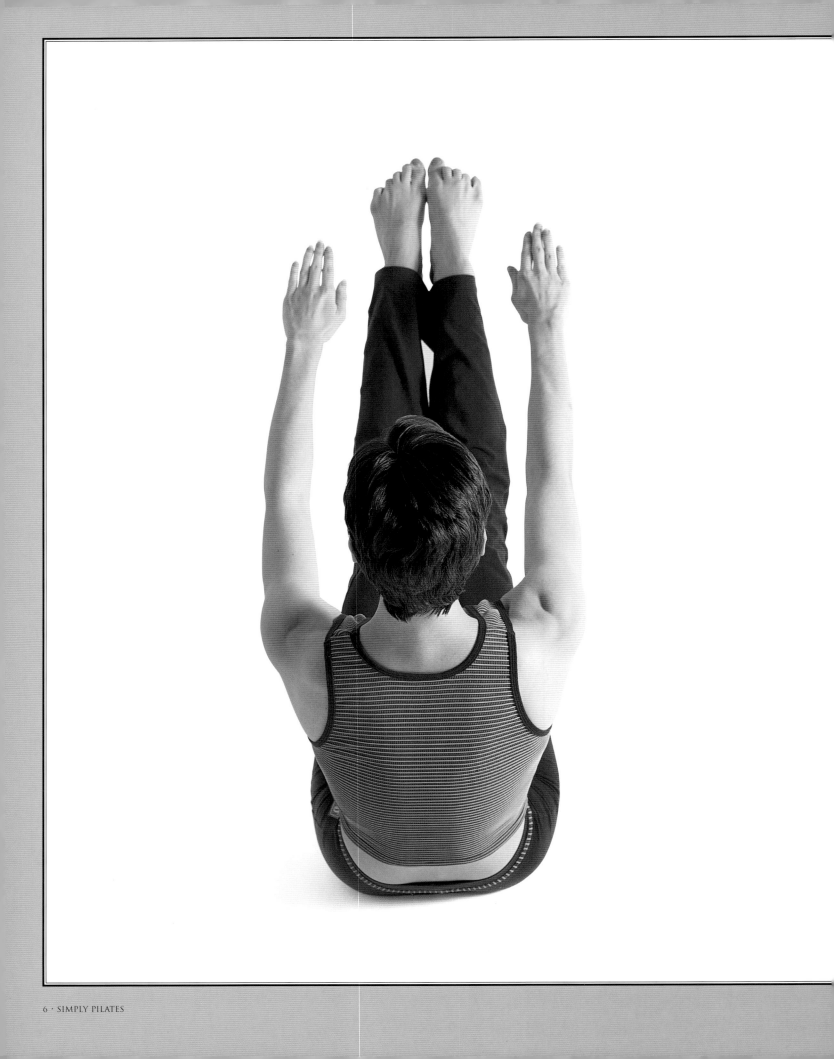

THE BENEFITS

A commitment to the Pilates mat work will promote greater trunk and pelvic stability, as well as improving movement and muscle control of and around the spine itself. Such control is requisite to both preventing spinal injury, and managing any existing back or neck pain. Pilates exercises specifically aim to create muscle balance in the body, greater coordination of movement and control of the abdominals and breathing. These exercises encourage the use of the body as a whole unit, developing strong, lean musculature, rather than allowing individual muscle groups to develop isolated strength and to become bulky. The philosophies behind the Pilates Method have been constant for many years, but it is only recently that people have begun to recognise its 'tried-and-true', more holistic approach to maintaining physical fitness.

The Pilates repertoire of exercises is very adaptable, with most exercises having both a modified and a progressive version. This is why Pilates can enable people of all fitness levels to enjoy its benefits. A typical Pilates mat work session will progress the exercises in a particular order, so that the muscles are prepared for subsequent exercises and a full-body workout is achieved. When these series of movements are executed in a precise and flowing manner, an authentic synergy between mind and body is met, natural poise is achieved, and overall well-being is enhanced.

Simply Pilates is a compilation of beginner-level exercises based on Joseph Pilates' original body-conditioning concepts. The sequence is designed to be easily interpreted for you to establish and maintain postural strength and balance. The Pilates way of exercising involves starting from basic awareness of your posture, movement and breathing. Once these essential concepts are embodied, you will find its benefits will translate to your everyday activities. Pilates will add to your enjoyment of life and assist you in reaching your fitness potential.

PRACTICAL MATTERS

When exercising the Pilates way, ensure that you are aware of the need to flatten your abdominals to stabilise your pelvis and lower back. If you have a history of injury, or physical limitation, or if you are pregnant, it is recommended that you consult your physician before embarking on any exercise program in order to assess the suitability of various movements for your body. Once you have received the all-clear, regular practice will help you to achieve your fitness goals more quickly, and will assist in the maintenance of optimum body balance. Three to four times a week is fine. Adapt the step-by-step directions to suit your physical capabilities and fitness level. The Pilates mat work is designed to allow you to proceed through the exercises at your own pace. Build up to the entire exercise program gradually, adding repetitions as you get stronger—though remember that 'less is more' and a maximum of 6–10 repetitions for each exercise is sufficient, providing each execution is of good quality.

REQUIREMENTS

You will need certain materials in order to do your Pilates mat work. The mat or carpet surface which you select must offer you some comfort, but must not be so soft that your body sinks into it and the natural curvature of your spine loses integrity. You will need a small pillow and a towel to assist with some exercises and stretches. You may also rest your head on either of these during the mat work if you need neck support. Finally, it is recommended that you use a low chair or box to relieve lower back tension during some sitting exercises.

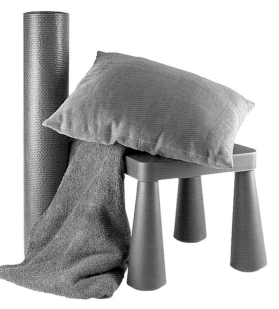

PILATES PRINCIPLES

There are six principles which help to define the purpose of the Pilates Method:

CONCENTRATION

The mind wills the body to perform. It is said that without mental focus during a workout, essentially only half a workout is being done. Visualisation assists the individual in using the correct muscles.

CONTROL

Pilates exercises require absolute muscle control to both guard against injury and to achieve full functional benefit from each movement.

CENTRE

The abdomen, lower back, hips and buttocks comprise our 'centre', the region which Joseph referred to as our 'powerhouse'—all energy for movement begins here, then continues to the extremities.

FLUIDITY

It is intended that the exercises be executed with optimal flow and grace. There are no static or isolated movements, and manoeuvres are never rushed.

PRECISION

Each movement has purpose and each repetition of an exercise is of high quality, so favourable muscle patterning will become second nature.

BREATH

Breathing with intention assists with muscle control. Inhaling and exhaling fully promotes purification and oxygenation of the lungs and bloodstream which energises the system and gives a feeling of well-being.

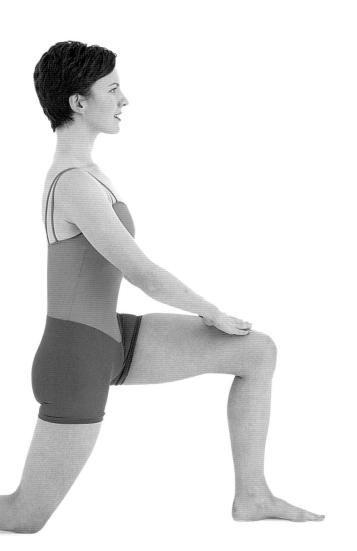

CENTRING & BREATHING

Each time you begin the Pilates mat work, be aware of the following important concepts, as they are fundamental in executing the exercises in their correct and intended form.

NEUTRAL PELVIS

The pelvis is the junction between the torso and legs, to which various muscles attach for movement and stabilising purposes. When the pelvis tilts forward or backward the curve of the lower back will change. Current spinal health research indicates that the natural curves of the spine should be maintained during exercise in order to strengthen the muscles essential to postural support. The correct positioning of the pelvis is crucial to maintaining this natural spinal shape. 'Neutral Pelvis' is achieved when the pelvic bones tilt neither way, but simply rest where hip and back muscles can remain fairly relaxed. The easiest way of finding this position is to recognise that your pubic bone and hip bones (iliac crests) all form a parallel level with the floor when lying on your back. (These bones should be aligned in the same plane when the body is in any position.) Neutral Pelvis is the ideal position in which to strengthen the deep abdominals.

CORRECT ABDOMINALS

Strong abdominals are more important to you than achieving a 'six-pack'. Good quality movement while preventing spinal injury begins by working the muscles from the inside out. This means refining the action of the abdominal muscles so that you can work the deeper layers responsible for maintaining 'core' stability. To target this area you need to focus on the 'drawing in and up' of the lower abdomen—between the pubic bone and navel. Imagine zipping up the abdominals starting from the pubic bone, as if you're zipping up tight jeans! Use pelvic floor muscles and flatten and tighten the abdominals towards the floor, without actually disturbing your Neutral Pelvis. Try not to tense up the gluteal muscles (buttocks). Imagine that your whole navel and waist area is shrinking, as though held in by a corset. During a Pilates session an instructor would typically describe this action as 'scooping', 'drawing in' or 'pressing the navel to spine' in order to ensure that the deeper layers of abdominals are strengthened.

BREATH CONTROL

Various breathing techniques are used for different purposes. Many people breathe insufficiently in order to nourish, energise and detoxify the body. Focusing on regular breathing when exercising is important, as oxygen is needed to assist in physical stamina, and breath monitoring helps to assist muscle use or relaxation. Breathe in through the nose and out through the mouth. Keep a steady pace, and ensure both the lower abdominals and the corset action of the waist remain active. When learning the Pilates Method of body conditioning, abdominal strength and control is a primary focus. Lateral, or sideways, breathing is taught so that the abdominal focus can remain strong. This is achieved when the side and back of the ribcage expand during inhalation and with each exhalation the abdominals 'scooping in and upward' is re-emphasised.

PREPARATORY NOTE

These posture cues are the basis of the Pilates Method. This specific attention to detail is imperative to both encourage correct use of muscles and to enable the release of muscles that have become overworked. Once this basis of functional posture is established, the Pilates exercises can be practised with a deeper understanding of restoring balance to the body. Attention must be paid to alignment of the body as a whole—from head to toes. To prepare for each exercise, the Neutral Pelvis Position should be established and the natural curves of the spine maintained, while ensuring the hip, knee and ankle joints are in line. The easiest way to align the legs is to place the heels opposite the 'sitting bones', which are the lowest bony protrusions of the pelvis that you may be aware of when sitting on a hard surface. Over time, constant awareness of good posture and muscular support will increase the endurance of the body's 'core' muscles. This will assist in the release of unnecessary tension and the management of aches and pains.

BREATHING EXERCISE

Purpose *To establish the basic postural concepts: maintaining a Neutral Pelvis Position while developing the coordination of lateral breathing with correct abdominal use. This technique of breathing and abdominal control is essentially how we begin every exercise. With practice it will gradually become second nature. Getting this correct will enable you to progress through the Pilates mat work and will challenge your strength, control and endurance.*

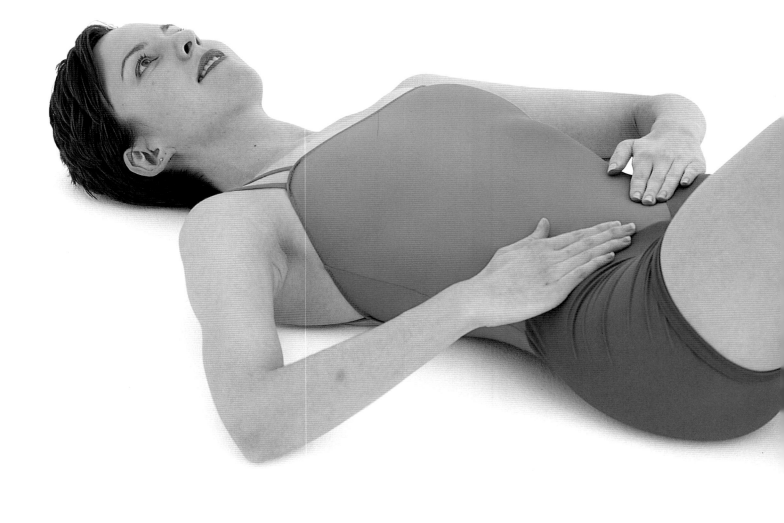

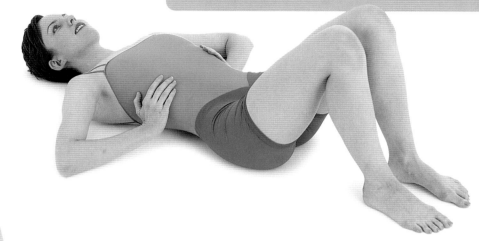

1 Lie on your back, with your knees bent, your heels opposite your sitting bones, and your hands resting on your lower abdomen. (We will refer to this as the 'Preparatory Position').

2 Inhale for the length of 4–5 counts, expanding through the side and back of your ribcage. The abdominals should remain controlled, drawing inward gently. The upper chest and neck should also remain fairly relaxed.

3 Exhale for the length of 4–5 counts, allowing your chest and ribs to fall while emphasising the drawing in of the lower abdominals. Use your pelvic floor muscles to create a deeper sensation of pelvic stability and control.

POSTURE AWARENESS & PELVIC STABILITY

Purpose *To challenge the ability to maintain a Neutral Pelvis Position and to develop abdominal and shoulder stability for postural endurance.*

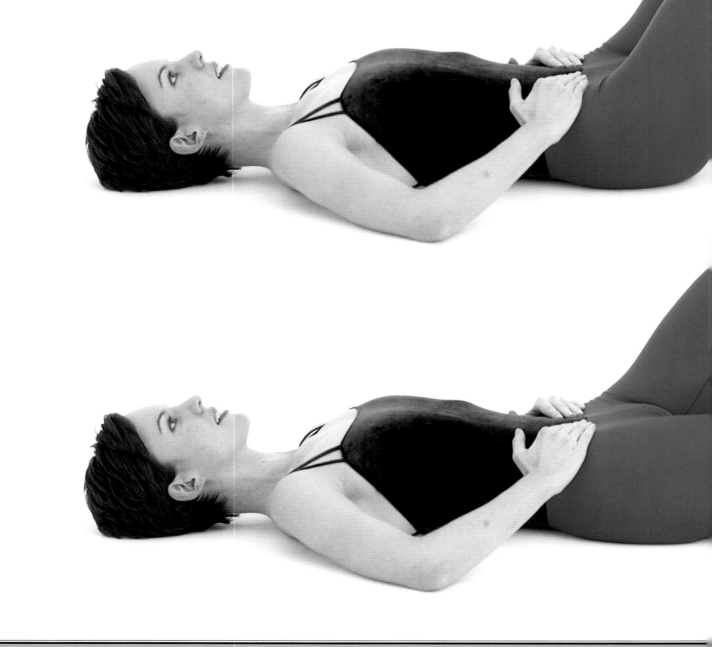

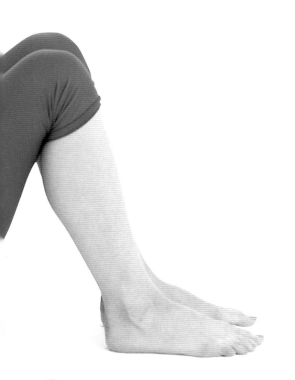

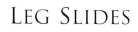

Leg Slides

1 Begin in the Preparatory Position, inhale in order to prepare, and then begin 'scooping' the abdominals (as was described in Centring and Breathing).

2 Exhale, sliding one heel along the floor, using your abdominals and maintaining control of your Neutral Pelvis Position.

3 Inhale, dragging the heel back to the Preparatory Position, always maintaining abdominal bracing and pelvic stability.

4 Repeat 10 times in all, alternating legs.

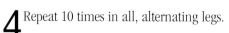

Posture Awareness
& Pelvic Stability

(continued)

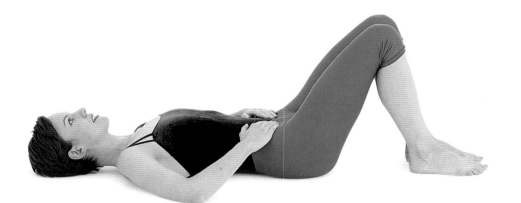

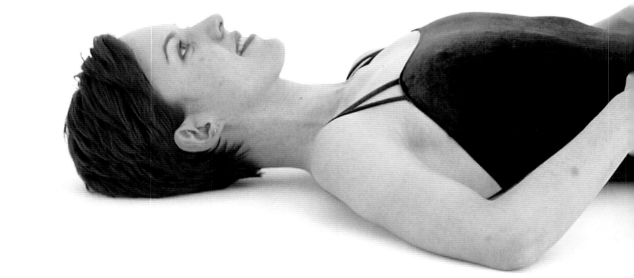

Leg Lifts

1 Begin in the Preparatory Position, and then begin scooping the abdominals.

2 Inhale as you lift your thigh towards the body so that your shin is parallel to the floor. Ensure deep abdominals and pelvic stability are your focus.

3 Exhale, lowering your foot back to the floor, maintaining control of your abdominals and Neutral Pelvis.

4 Repeat 10 times in all, alternating legs.

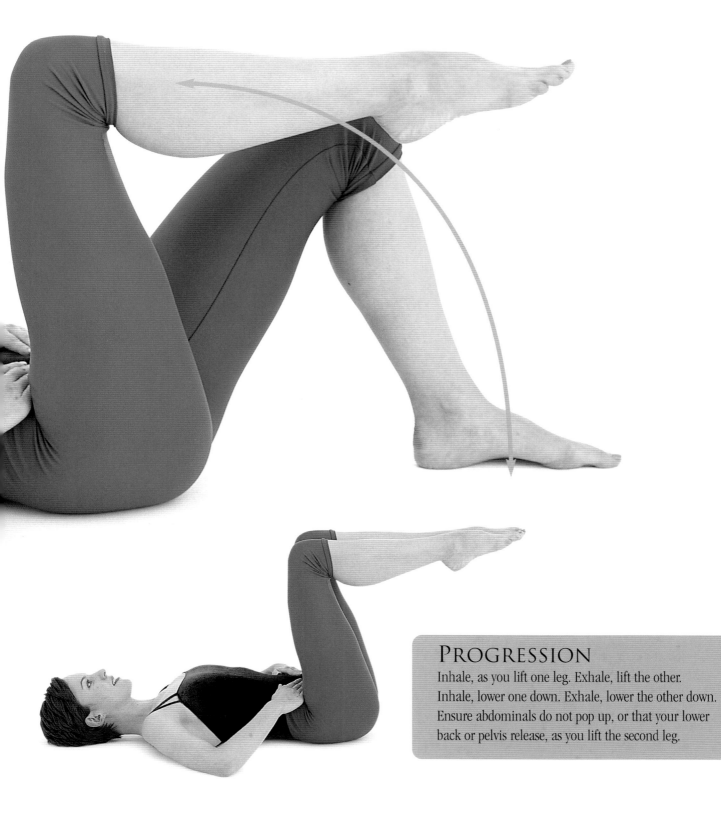

PROGRESSION

Inhale, as you lift one leg. Exhale, lift the other. Inhale, lower one down. Exhale, lower the other down. Ensure abdominals do not pop up, or that your lower back or pelvis release, as you lift the second leg.

POSTURE AWARENESS
& PELVIC STABILITY

(continued)

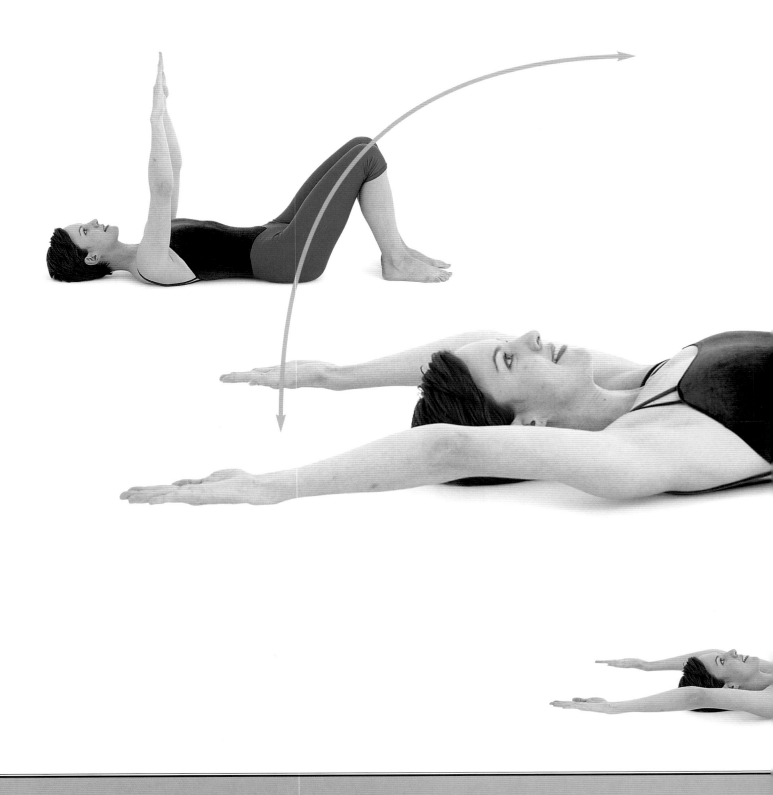

SHOULDER STABILITY

1 Begin in the Preparatory Position. Reach your arms towards the ceiling, with your shoulders drawing down.

2 Inhale to reach your arms over your head, maintaining your natural spinal position. Be careful not to allow your ribs to lose contact with the floor, or your shoulders to shrug upward.

3 Exhale, bringing your arms back towards the ceiling, emphasising your shoulders drawing down against the floor, and bracing your abdominals.

4 Repeat 4–6 times, for general awareness of shoulder stability and coordination of abdominal and breath control.

PROGRESSION

To challenge your coordination, combine the Leg Slides and Shoulder Stability exercises. Inhale to slide your heel down as your arms reach overhead. Exhale to pull your leg and arms back to the Preparatory Position. Focus on abdominals and drawing your shoulders down, with no movement of the spine or pelvis.

Spinal
Mobility

Purpose *Abdominal preparation, developing fluid spinal motion, and strengthening back, gluteals and hips.*

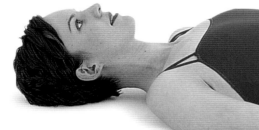

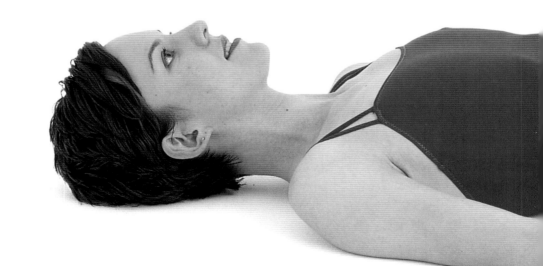

PELVIC TILT

1 Begin in the Preparatory Position, with your arms relaxed.
Inhale laterally and begin scooping your abdominals.

2 Exhale, drawing your lower abdominals inward to initiate
a pelvic tilt backward, stretching your lower back. Make
sure that your buttocks are relaxed and your feet are firmly
planted on the floor.

3 Inhale to roll your pelvis back to Neutral, and relax your
hips completely.

4 Repeat 4–5 times.

SPINAL MOBILITY

(continued)

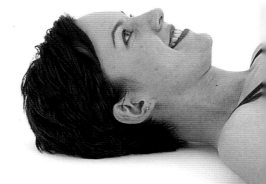

PELVIC CURL

1 Begin as for the Pelvic Tilt.

2 Exhale, scooping your lower abdominals to initiate a pelvic tilt backward, and roll your spine off the floor, aiming to articulate each segment. Use the muscles beneath your buttocks to lift your pelvis to eliminate any possibility of back strain.

3 Inhale laterally, maintaining this position. Keep your feet firmly on the floor, your thighs parallel and neck and shoulders relaxed.

4 Exhale, rolling the spine down to the floor with control. Maintain leg alignment and imagine lengthening the spine as it rolls.

5 Inhale as you relax your hips completely.

6 Repeat 5–6 times.

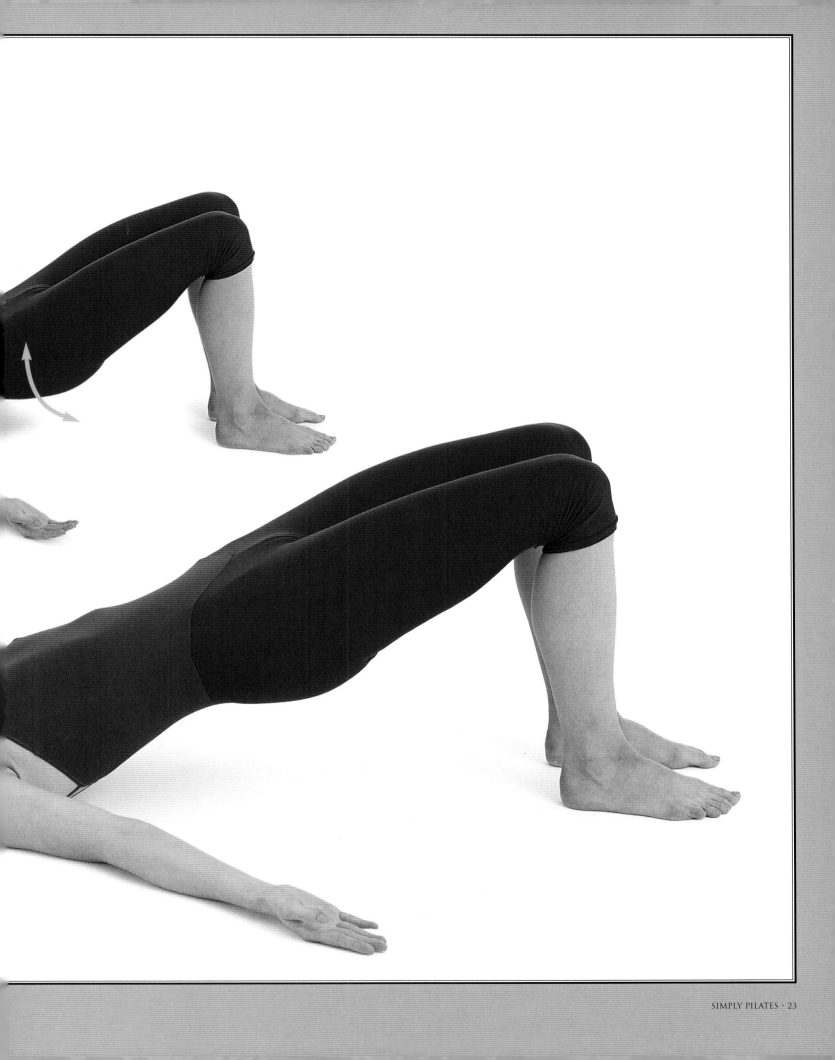

SPINAL MOBILITY

(continued)

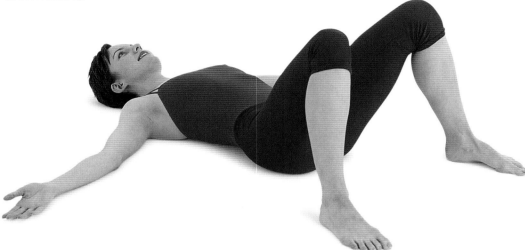

KNEES SIDE-TO-SIDE

1 Part your feet until they are slightly wider than your pelvis, and prepare your abdominals.

2 Inhale as you allow your thighs to gently fall to one side, causing the pelvis to roll sideways. Keep your shoulder blades on the floor.

3 Emphasise your abdominals, exhaling as you roll the pelvis back to Neutral, with the legs following.

4 Repeat 6–10 times in all, alternating sides.

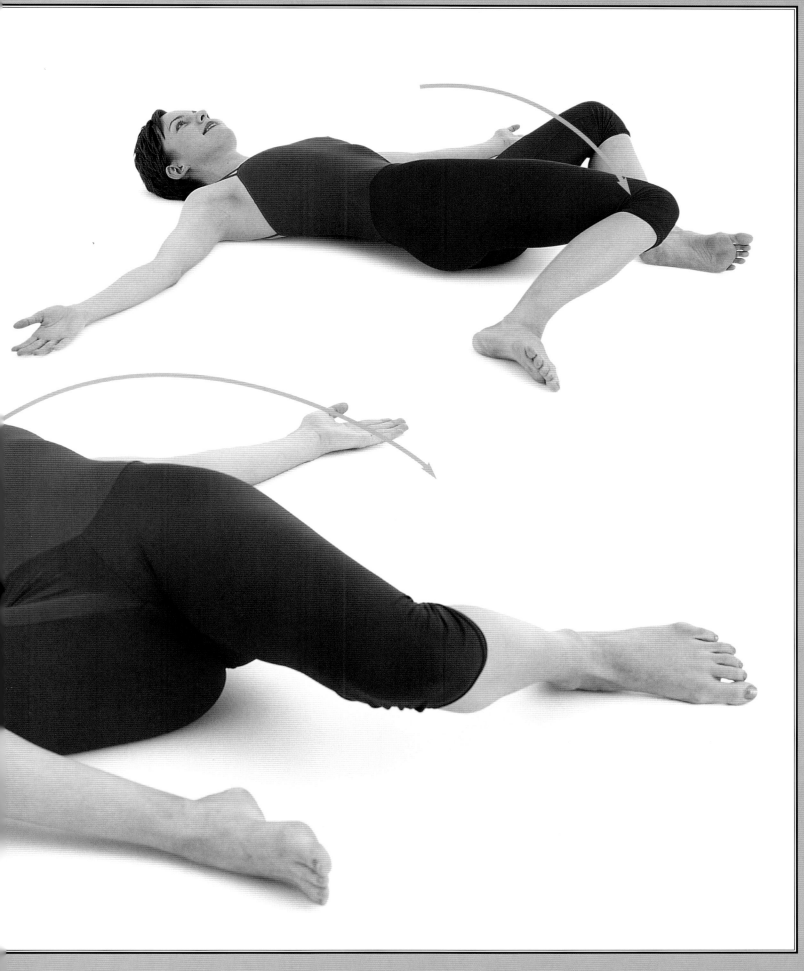

ABDOMINAL WARM-UP

Purpose *Gentle abdominal work and developing breath control, while focusing on pelvic stability and leg alignment. These exercises are a preparation for subsequent exercises.*

CHEST LIFT

1 Begin in the Preparatory Position, with your hands behind your neck.

2 Prepare by inhaling and scooping your abdominals.

3 Exhale, lifting your head, neck and shoulders off the floor, pressing the abdominals towards your spine. Maintain Neutral Pelvis and resist overusing back, leg and gluteal muscles.

4 Inhale laterally, maintaining abdominal flattening and chest height.

5 Exhale, lowering your head and shoulders, and maintaining your abdominal scooping.

6 Repeat 5–6 times.

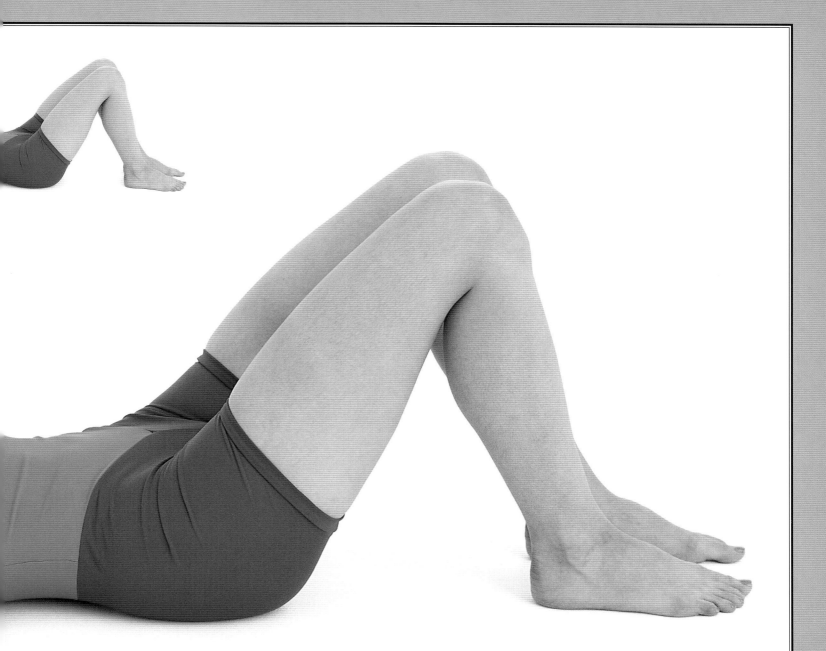

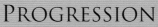

PROGRESSION

After 5–6 repetitions, repeat with leg lifts. Hold the Chest Lift position, and inhale as you lift one thigh, exhale as you lower your foot to the floor. Repeat with your other leg, then inhale to hold and maintain your abdominal scooping and exhale as you lower your head and shoulders.

ABDOMINAL WARM-UP

(continued)

HUNDREDS PREP

1 Begin with your knees directly over your hips, with shins
parallel to the floor. (We will refer to this position of the
legs as 'Tabletop Position'.) Hands are on your knees,
abdominals are drawing in and shoulders are drawing down.
Then, inhale to prepare.

2 Exhale to emphasise abdominal scooping as the head and
shoulders lift, reaching the arms down past your hips. Do
not lose control of the Neutral Pelvis Position, or allow your
stomach to pop up.

3 Inhale laterally, as you lower your head and shoulders
while maintaining abdominal control. Bring your hands
back to your knees.

4 Repeat 5–6 times.

If your abdominals are weak, or you experience back
pain, rest your feet on a chair while curling up and
down. Alternatively, your physician may recommend
that you do not execute any exercises where both legs
are in the air.

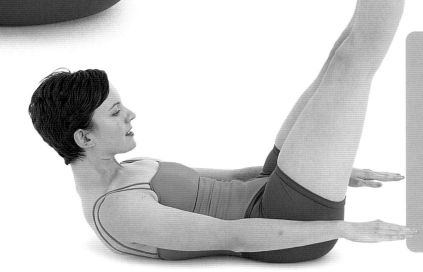

PROGRESSION

Once you are achieving a curl and maintaining absolute pelvic stability and flat abdominals, try extending your legs upward as you curl and reach both arms down by your sides. Bend your knees fractionally before lowering the head and shoulders to protect your back from arching off the floor.

ABDOMINAL WARM-UP

(continued)

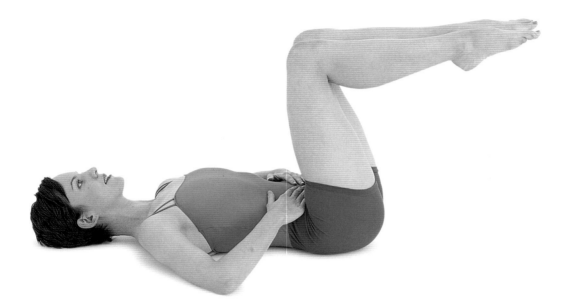

HUNDREDS

1 Begin as we did for the Breathing Exercise. There are a few progressions from the basic breathing to challenge your abdominal and breath control.

2 If you can maintain correct abdominal flattening and have no back pain, raise your legs to the Tabletop Position and repeat the breathing (4–5 counts in, 4–5 counts out). If this is too difficult, rest your heels on a chair to help support the weight of your legs.

3 *Next progression*—maintaining the legs at Tabletop, lift your head and shoulders and reach both arms down by your hips. Continue the same breathing pattern and use small arm movements (pulsing up and down) to maintain a rhythm for your breath and counting. Build up to 10 full breaths in this manner, as you develop greater abdominal stamina and control.

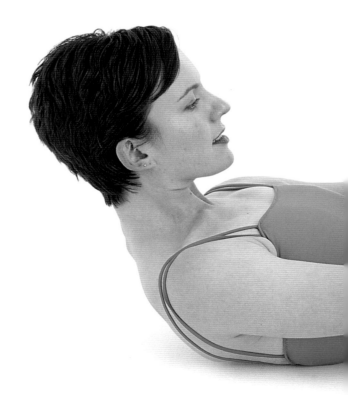

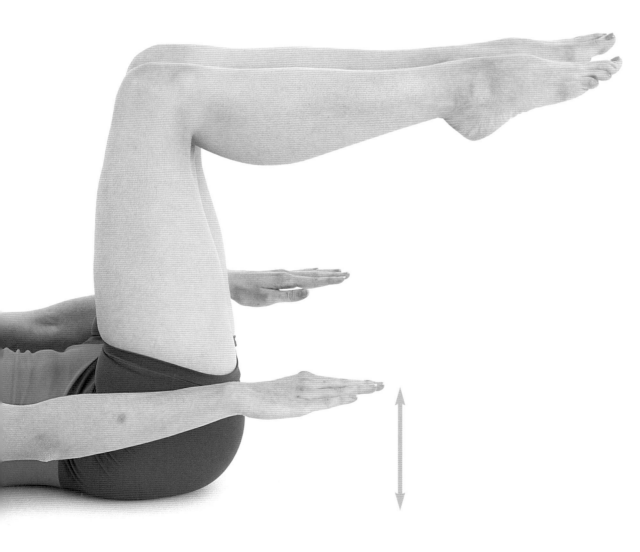

PROGRESSION

Step 3 is a classic Pilates exercise known as Hundreds. As you gain strength, extend your legs toward the ceiling and slightly away from you. Remember to keep scooping your abdominals and maintain a stable Neutral Pelvis Position. Don't progress yourself to the extended leg position until you are ready.

ABDOMINAL WARM-UP

(continued)

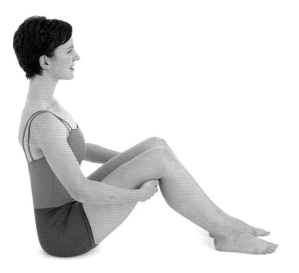

ROLL UP PREP

1 Start in a seated position, with your legs bent in front of you and slightly apart. Hold your hands gently beneath your knees. Sit up straight with your shoulders down and abdominals scooping in and upward, and then inhale to prepare.

2 Exhale, pulling your navel toward your spine to initiate a pelvic tilt backward so that you can roll back sufficiently to challenge the abdominals—without losing the round lower back position. Ensure that the abdominals are working, and not the legs or arms!

3 Inhale laterally, to hold still, deepening the abdominals without other physical tensions.

4 Exhale to roll forward to resume the seated position. Again, ensure that it is actually the abdominals that move you.

5 Repeat 6–10 times, being careful to roll only to a position in which you can maintain full abdominal control.

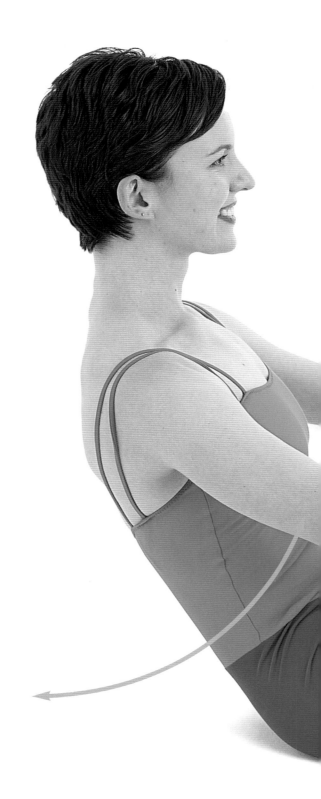

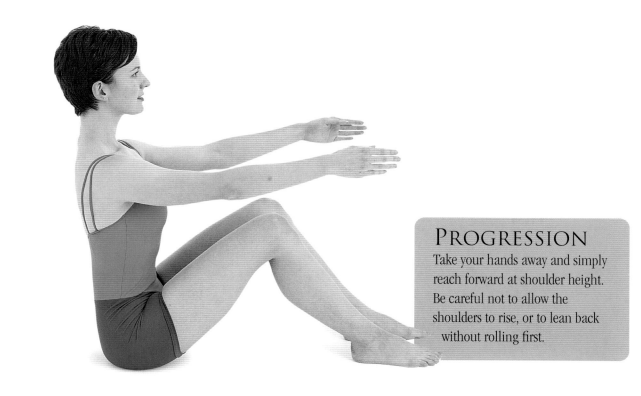

PROGRESSION

Take your hands away and simply reach forward at shoulder height. Be careful not to allow the shoulders to rise, or to lean back without rolling first.

ABDOMINAL STRENGTHENING

Purpose *To further challenge the abdominals and the stability of the pelvis while limbs or upper torso are moving.*

OBLIQUE LIFTS

1 Begin in the Preparatory Position, with your hands behind your head and neck. Then, inhale to prepare.

2 Exhale as the head and shoulders lift, rotating your upper torso and pressing the abdominals down to establish a strong position of the pelvis and waistline. Your pelvis and legs should not move.

3 Inhale as you lower back to the floor. Maintain your abdominal scooping action and imagine lengthening your spine.

4 Repeat 8–10 times, alternating sides.

NOTE
Be careful not to fold the arms in around your head. Instead, twist your body so that the shoulder aims in the direction of the opposite knee, while the underneath shoulder blade gently presses against the floor.

ABDOMINAL STRENGTHENING

(continued)

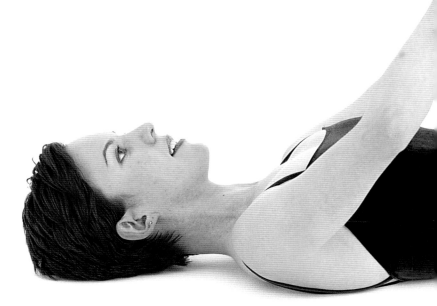

SINGLE LEG STRETCH

1 Lie on your back, with your legs in the Tabletop Position and hands on your knees. Inhale to prepare and start scooping the abdominals.

2 Exhale as one leg extends upward and away from your body, maintaining abdominals and drawing your shoulders down.

3 Inhale as you draw the leg back. Try to emphasise scooping your abdominals on each inhalation, as this is the preparation for the next leg extension!

4 Exhale as you extend the other leg.

5 Repeat 8–10 times, alternating legs.

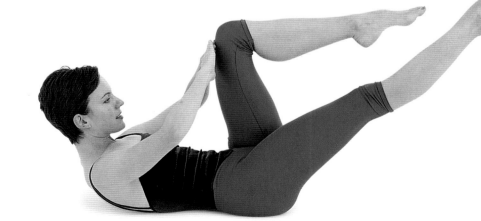

PROGRESSION

For additional abdominal work, curl your head and shoulders off the floor throughout.

SPINAL ROTATION

Purpose *To encourage correct muscular support as the spine executes a rotatory movement, while managing pelvic and shoulder girdle stability.*

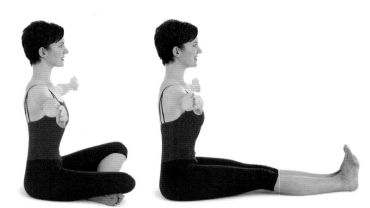

SPINE TWIST

1 Sit tall, with both legs either extended straight out in front of your body, or crossed. (This depends on deciding which is the best position for you to sit in without slumping in the lower back. A small box or chair may be needed to relieve pressure on your lower back, enabling this upright posture.)

2 Extend your arms sideways at shoulder height, palms turned backward and shoulders drawing down. Anchor your hips to the floor, and if the legs are straight in front, bring your knees and ankles firmly together. This will help maintain your sense of pelvic stability.

3 Inhale to 'grow' tall, abdominals drawing in and upward, shoulders down.

4 Exhale as you twist from the waist with a double pulse action. Ensure that your hips don't rotate or lift, and that your shoulders don't rise or drop on one side! Imagine spiralling the spine upwards.

5 Inhale as you return to the centre, maintaining a tall seated position. Remember to breathe laterally and to keep drawing your abdominals in and upward.

6 Repeat 8–10 times, alternating sides.

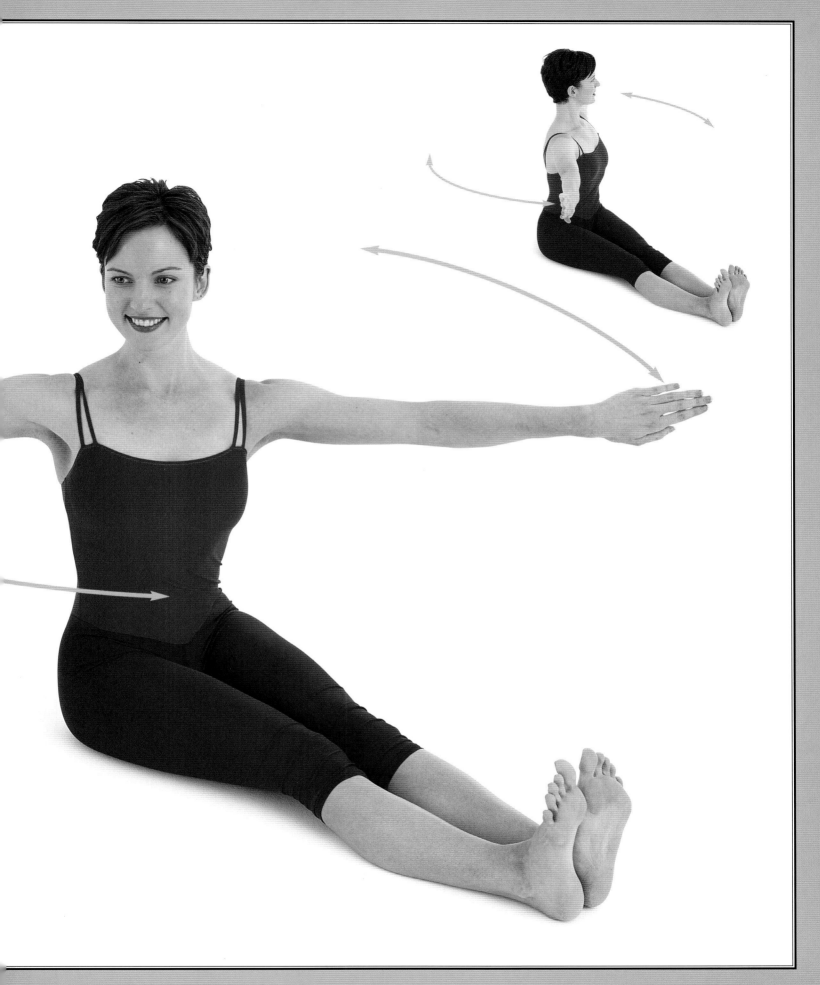

Side Stability, Gluteals & Inside Thighs

Purpose *Strengthening of the side, hip and inside thigh muscles, while still maintaining abdominal and postural support. Since it's more difficult to balance when lying on the side, this is also a position which is useful to challenge and develop spinal and pelvic stability.*

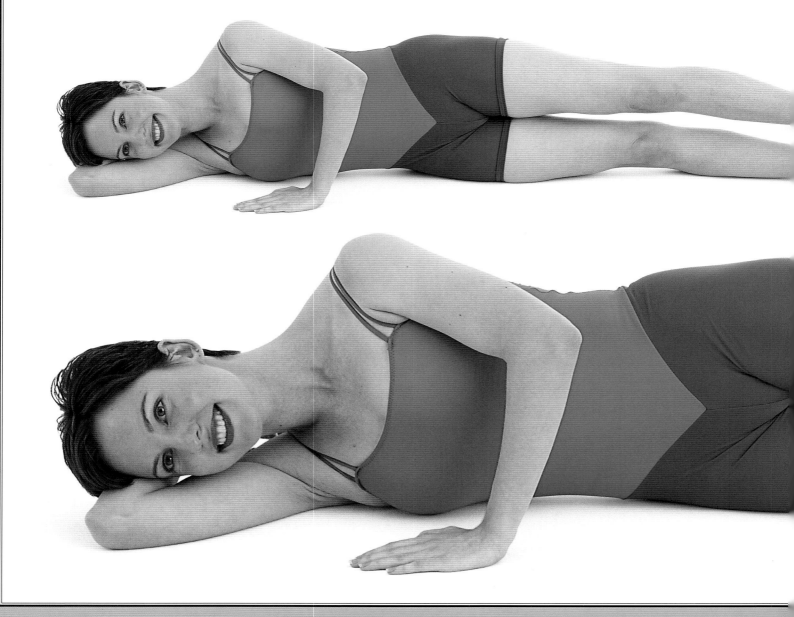

SIDE LEG LIFTS

1 Lie on one side with both legs extending longways and slightly forward of your body. When on the side, one hip bone should be directly vertically aligned with the other. Place the hand of your top arm on the floor in front of your torso— this is a gentle reminder to use the abdominals to stabilise you, and is not there to prop you up!

2 Inhale to prepare and stabilise your torso with the abdominals.

3 Exhale, lengthening both legs away and lifting them just clear of the floor.

4 Inhale as you lower them.

5 Repeat 10 times, each side, ensuring that your lower back doesn't arch or strain.

NOTE
If this is too difficult, or if back pain is experienced, start by lifting only your top leg a few inches and maintaining focus on your abdominals for side balancing.

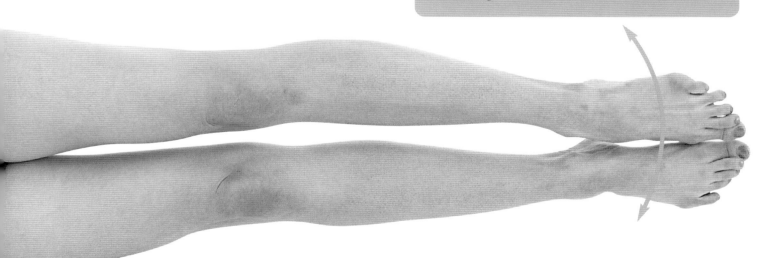

SIDE STABILITY, GLUTEALS
& INSIDE THIGHS

(continued)

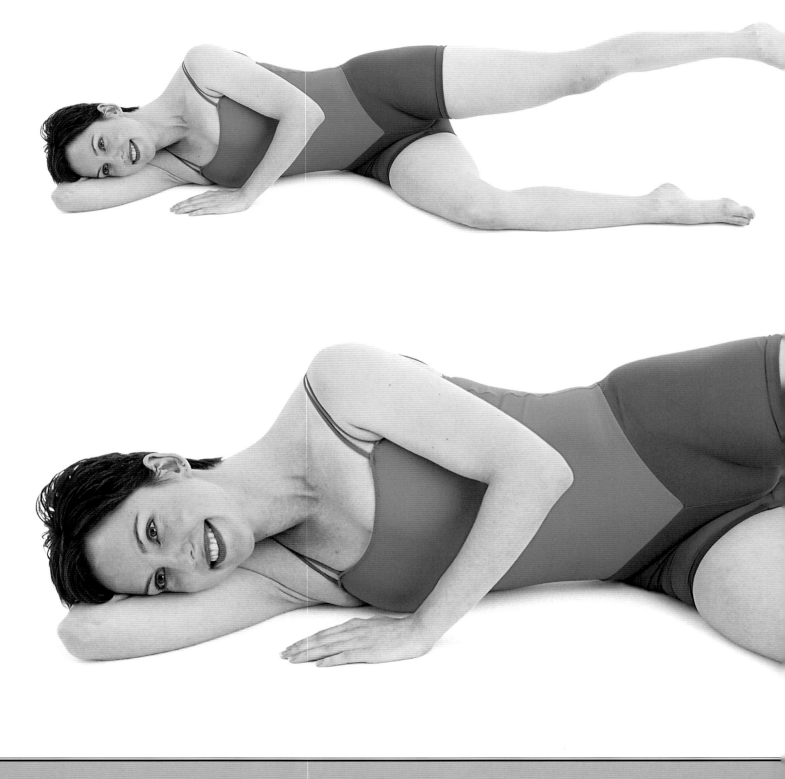

WALL GLUTES

1 Lie on one side, as if your torso were against a wall. Maintain all the crucial curves of the spine and place your underneath leg forward of your body, bent, for stability. Your top leg is extended longways, though not rigid. Your thigh should relax inward slightly.

2 Exhale as you lift your leg slightly and hold momentarily. Maintain absolute pelvic stability, lifting predominately from the back of your hip.

3 Inhale as you slowly lower your leg.

4 Repeat 10–15 times each side.

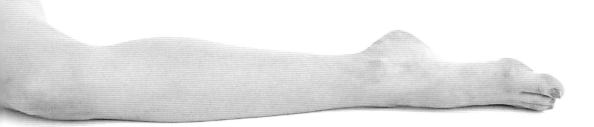

SIDE STABILITY, GLUTEALS & INSIDE THIGHS

(continued)

CUSHION SQUEEZE

1 Begin in the Preparatory Position, with a cushion placed between your thighs. Inhale to prepare the abdominals.

2 Exhale as you emphasise your abdominals drawing in and upward and squeeze your thighs together. Focus on abdominals and inside thighs—keep your gluteal muscles fairly relaxed, and ensure a Neutral Pelvis Position is maintained.

3 Inhale as you hold the squeeze, maintaining abdominals.

4 Exhale as you release the cushion.

5 Repeat 8–10 times.

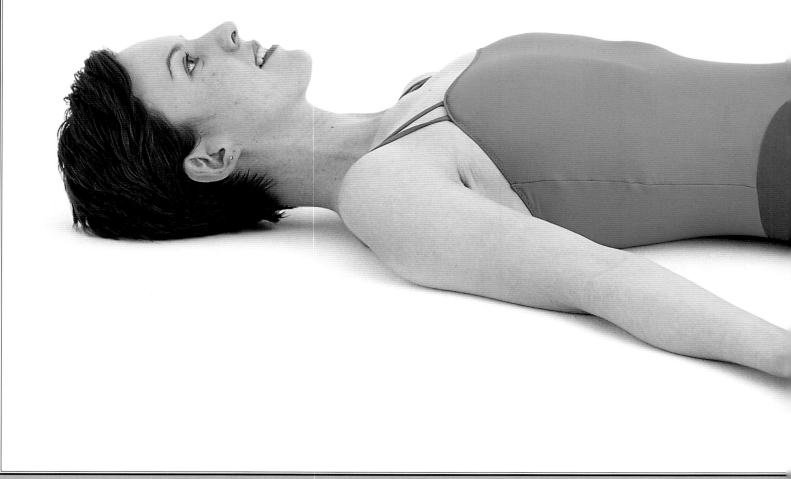

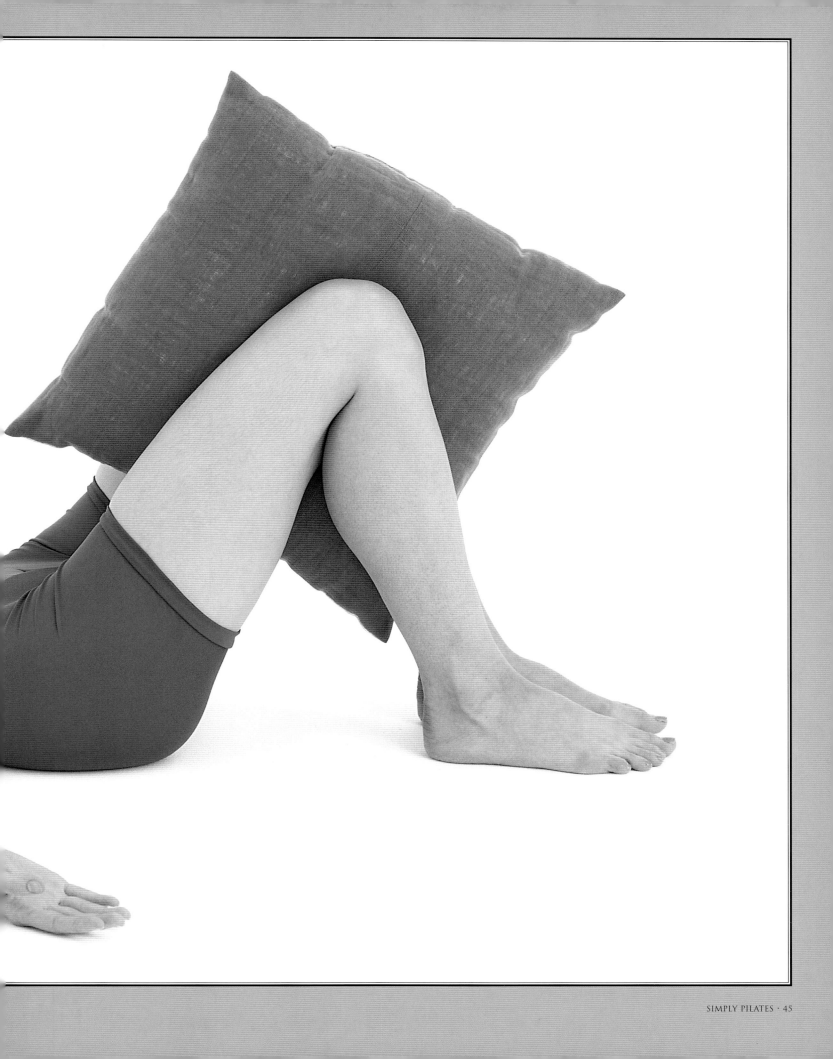

SCAPULA STABILITY & BACK STRENGTHENING

Purpose *Correct scapula (shoulder blade) and shoulder positioning is necessary to develop endurance of the postural muscles. When the middle and upper back become stronger, stress is reduced for the neck and shoulder joints.*

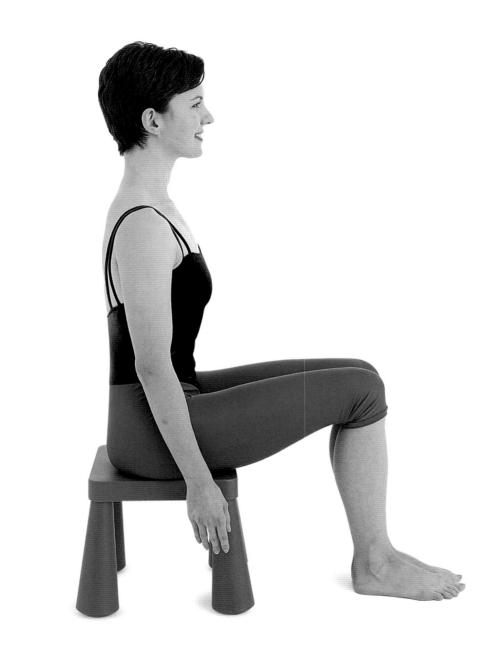

Arm raises (front & side)

1 Begin sitting or standing. Lengthen your spine, draw abdominals in and upward and gently pull your shoulders back to broaden the chest. Start with your arms relaxed by your sides, with the palms of your hands facing the body.

2 Inhale, raising your arms forward while maintaining the shoulder blades in a flat position. Only raise your arms to a height where the shoulder blades don't protrude, or 'wing', and the shoulders don't shrug upward.

3 Exhale as you lower your arms.

4 Repeat 8–10 times.

Scapula Stability & Back Strengthening

(continued)

Arm Raises (continued)

5 Repeat with your arms lifting sideways, though slightly forward of your torso. Palms of the hands should now be facing the front, and your shoulder blades should still remain flat. Ensuring that the abdominals still draw in and upward, keep a sense of length through the waist, and calmness in the neck and upper chest. Imagine a trickle of water running down the centre of your upper back. A feeling of strength and bracing should be felt there.

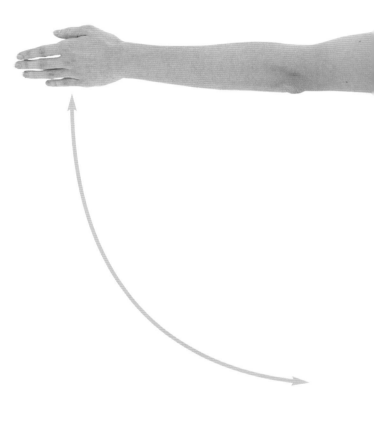

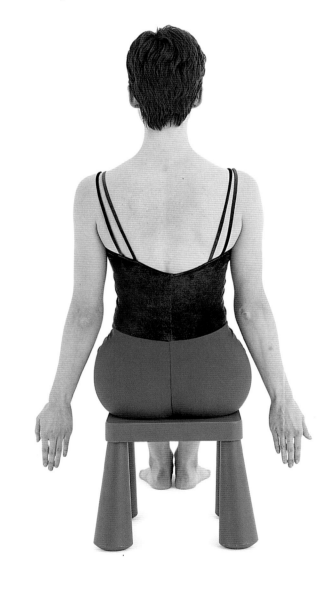

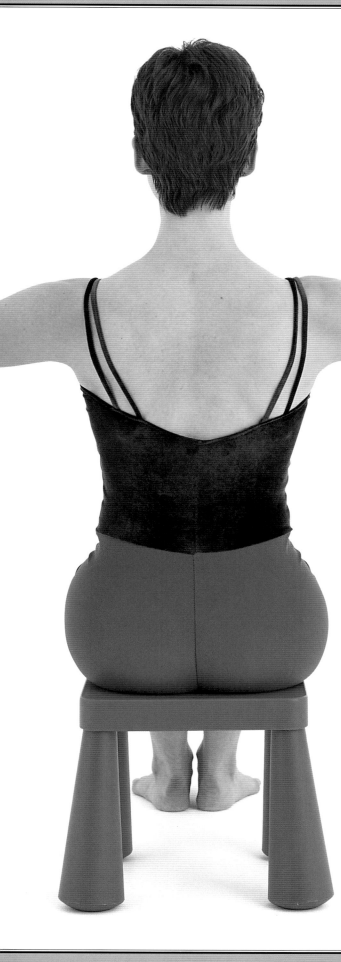

NOTE

It may be beneficial to lean against a wall in order to feel the sensation of keeping the scapulae completely flat against a hard surface.

PROGRESSION

Once scapula stability is achieved, a light weight of a kilo or half a kilo may be added to each hand for the purpose of further strengthening.

SCAPULA STABILITY & BACK STRENGTHENING

(continued)

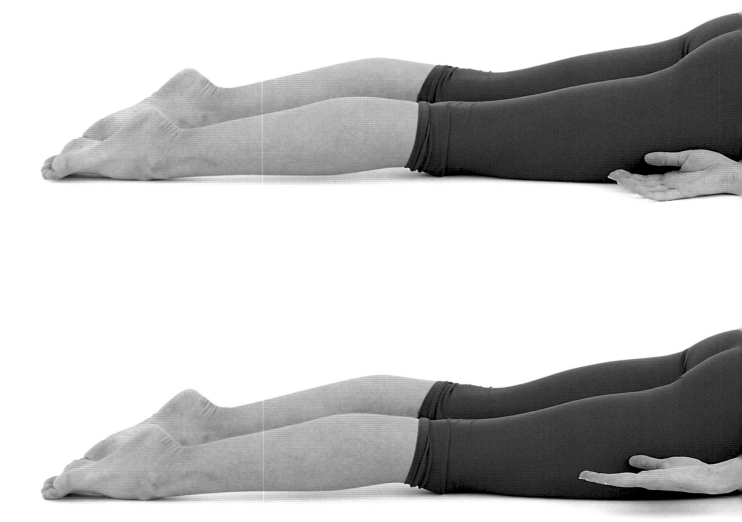

BACK EXTENSION

1 Lie face down, arms beside your body and forehead resting on a small cushion, or rolled towel. Without altering your natural back position, draw your lower abdominals deep up toward the spine. Inhale to prepare.

2 Exhale, drawing the shoulders and hands back as if pressing against a wall when standing. Maintain your abdominals and upper back 'bracing' while keeping the chest and ribs on the floor (head and shoulders 'hover' off the floor).

3 Inhale, holding this position. Keep your nose pointing toward the floor so that your neck remains in line with the rest of the spine. Maintain abdominals. Reach toward the toes.

4 Exhale as you rest.

5 Repeat 8–10 times.

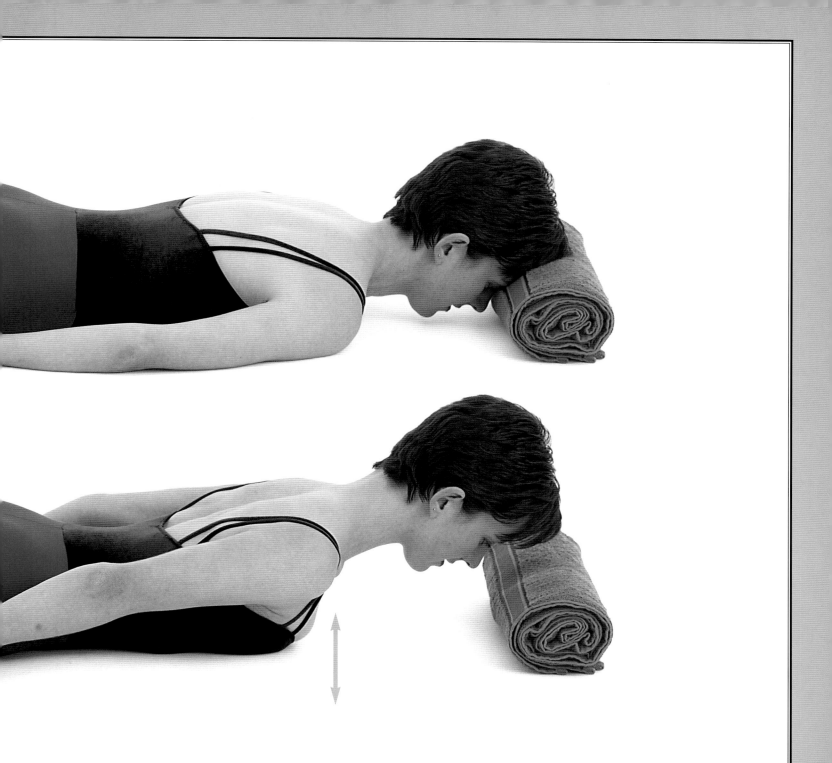

FULL BODY INTEGRATION

Purpose *Here are a couple of preparations for some full-body challenges, the Pilates way. Relying on the deep abdominals, back and hip muscles, these two exercises are primers for movement that requires abdominal strength flexibility and muscle control.*

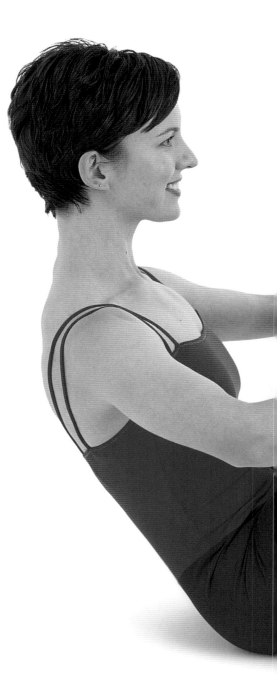

TEASER PREP BALANCE

1 Begin in a sitting position, with your knees bent, your hands under the thighs and feet lightly placed on the floor.

2 Roll back onto your tailbone and stabilise the position with your abdominals. Your feet should hover just off the floor, as you maintain abdominals and try to limit muscle tension in the thighs. Shoulders are relaxed.

3 Focus on breathing naturally and laterally. Keep scooping your abdominals and maintain a constant distance between the chest and knees.

4 Maintain this position, while breathing, for 6–8 breaths.

5 On the next inhalation, raise your shins so they become parallel with the floor—not allowing your torso or thigh position to change. More abdominals!

6 Exhale as you control the lowering of your shins.

7 Repeat 6–8 times.

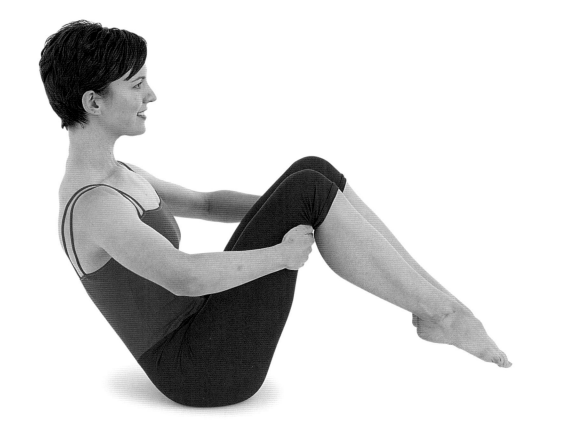

FULL BODY INTEGRATION

(continued)

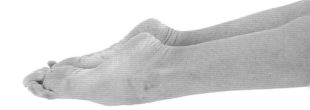

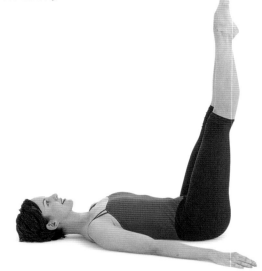

ROLL OVERS

1 Lie on your back, with your legs together and stretched toward the ceiling, and your arms by your sides. Inhale to prepare the abdominals. Depending on your hamstring flexibility, you may need to bend your knees a little.

2 Exhale as you use the abdominals strongly to lift your legs and hips up and over your head. Ensure that you don't strain with your neck, shoulders and arms. Abdominals should not pop out.

3 Inhale as you flex your feet and separate them to shoulder width while your legs remain parallel to the floor.

4 Exhale, rolling through your spine one vertebra at a time, abdominals controlling the movement. Your neck and shoulders should be as relaxed as possible.

5 Finish the roll, returning the pelvis back to Neutral and then inhale as the legs come back together, stretch them to the ceiling, and prepare to repeat.

6 Repeat 5–6 times.

> ### NOTE
> This exercise is unsuitable for people with neck or lower back injuries.

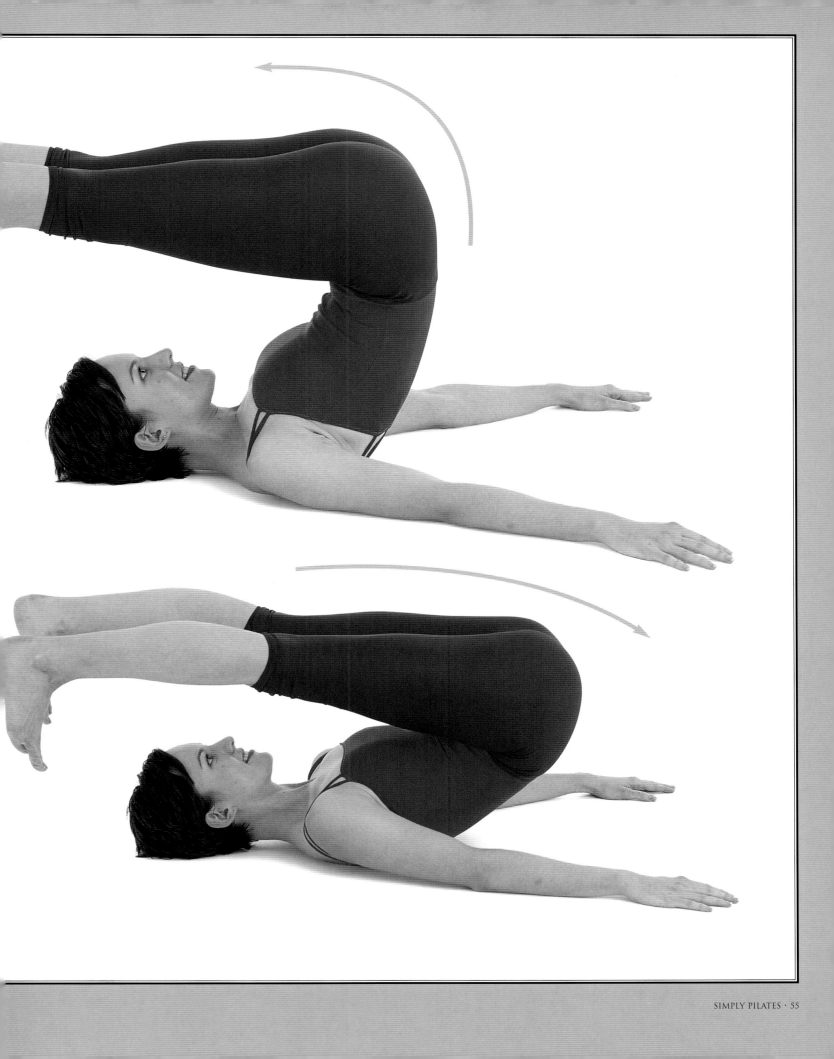

Stretches

Purpose *During and following muscle work, stretching helps muscles recover. There is also a definite need to develop a balance of strength with flexibility in order to reduce the risk of injury or strain. Lengthened muscles have the capacity to gain more strength and create a lithe, streamlined physique.*

Note

All stretches are to be held for 3–4 breaths to allow the muscles time to relax. Repeat for the other side, then repeat both sides again. If unnecessary strain is present, reduce or stop the stretch and consult your physician.

HAMSTRINGS

Lie on your back holding a towel around one foot, and the other leg stretched along the floor. Maintain a Neutral Pelvis Position and gently pull the raised leg toward you, aiming your heel toward the ceiling.

STRETCHES

(continued)

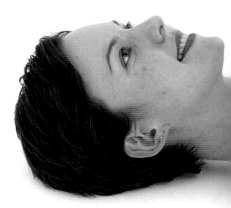

QUADRICEPS

Lie on your side, with your underneath knee bent and
pulled up toward your chest. Hold the foot of the top leg
behind you, with your thigh parallel to the floor. Pull your
foot to achieve a stretch at the front of your thigh. Gently push
the top hip forward as you pull your thigh back. Brace with
the abdominals.

GLUTEALS (BUTTOCKS)

Lying on your back, cross one ankle over the other knee and pull both legs toward you, ensuring that your tailbone does not leave the floor. Keep your hips as square as possible, and relax the hip muscles.

STRETCHES

(continued)

HIP FLEXORS

Kneel on one knee with the other leg bent and in front of your body. Both legs should remain aligned with the hips, with both hip bones facing front. Draw your abdominals in and upward, tilting the pelvis backward (as you did in the Pelvic Curl exercise) and lean slightly forward—resist sinking into your lower back, but keep 'zipping up' the abdominals and the front of the stretching hip.

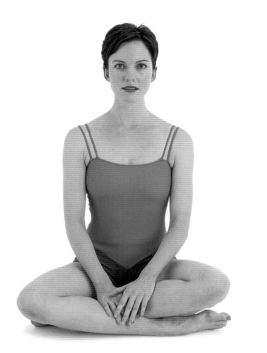
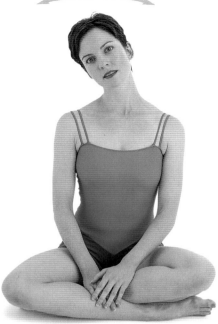
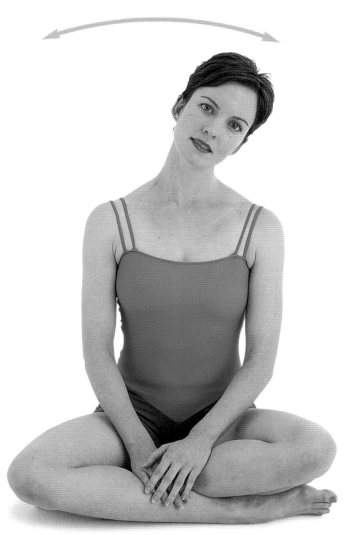

NECK

Sit, comfortably, with upright posture. Allow your head to tilt directly to one side—'ear to shoulder'. The opposite shoulder gently pulls downward.

GLOSSARY FOR MUSCLE TERMINOLOGY

GLUTEALS

Muscle group of the buttocks, that contribute to hip movement and pelvic/back stability.

HAMSTRINGS

Muscle group of the back of the thigh, from the hip to the knee, that bend the knee or assist in backward leg motion.

HIP FLEXORS

Muscles at the front of the hip that lift the thigh towards the torso.

OBLIQUE ABDOMINALS

The side muscles of the abdomen that twist, or rotate, the torso.

QUADRICEPS

Muscle group of the front of the thigh, from the hip to the knee, that makes up the major muscle mass of the thigh.

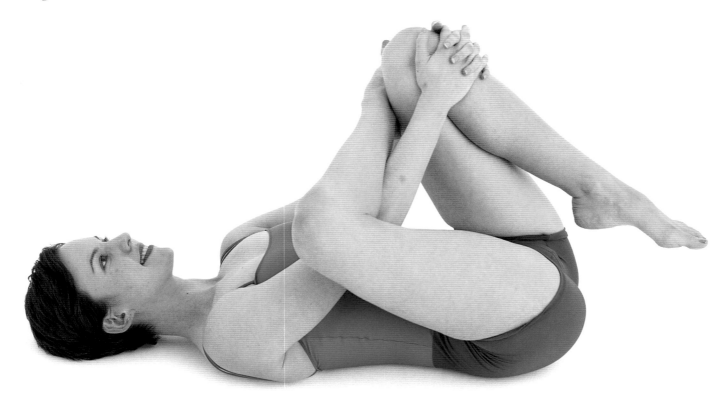

CONCLUSION

The Pilates Method has emerged from various philosophies that endorse physical health and longevity. This technique of conditioning the body and mind was developed with the intention to re-create an individual's approach to exercise and fitness in general. Far beyond the 'no pain, no gain' mentality of working the body, Pilates enforces muscle control and endurance without resulting in post-exercise soreness and fatigue. This method is suitable for all ages and levels of fitness. It incorporates all the essential concepts in order to achieve postural and lifestyle improvements and sports-specific cross-training benefits and provides a way in which to learn about your body and develop greater levels of agility, energy and concentration.

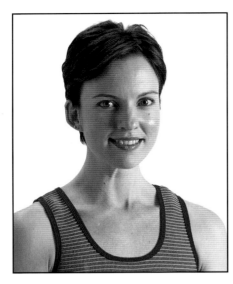

ABOUT THE AUTHOR

JENNIFER POHLMAN
completed a Bachelor of Dance
at the Victorian College of the
Arts in Melbourne and has
several years experience with
the Pilates Method. She began
Pilates training first as a dancer,
as a rehabilitative measure for
chronic lower back injury. This
progressed to instructor training
by means of an apprentice-
based course over an intensive
six-month period. While
teaching for over two years in
busy Brisbane and Gold Coast
studios, she established her
own business 'Pilates
InsideOut'. Jennifer teaches and
freelances in the Tweed River
and Gold Coast areas. Her
approach to the Pilates Method
is both dynamic and innovative
and she is experienced with
clients of all fitness levels and
ages—from athletes to clinical
rehabilitation patients.